THE FOUR PILLARS
OF
CELLULAR HEALTH

RICK BINDER

THE FOUR PILLARS
OF
CELLULAR HEALTH

RICK BINDER

ISBN-13: 978-1530080366
ISBN-10: 1530080363

Rick Binder

PO Box 22735

San Diego, CA 92192

(858) 707-5606

Rabinder2006@gmail.com

www.AnythingIsPossibleFitness.com

Medical Disclaimer

Always consult your physician before beginning any exercise program. This general information is not intended to diagnose any medical condition or to replace your healthcare professional. Consult with your healthcare professional to design an appropriate exercise prescription. If you experience any pain or difficulty with these exercises, stop and consult your healthcare provider. If you experience any symptoms of weakness, unsteadiness, light-headedness or dizziness, chest pain or pressure, nausea, or shortness of breath. Mild soreness after exercise may be experienced after beginning a new exercise. Contact your physician if the soreness does not improve after 3-4 days

The information contained in this book has not been evaluated by the Food and Drug Administration (FDA). The Information found on this website should not be used to diagnose, cure, prevent or mitigate disease. This website is provided for educational purposes only. Statements contained herein are presented in an effort to share information about free radical biology , medicinal foods and advances in nutrition only. Content may change frequently and may be incomplete; consequently, information presented herein may not be accurate until finalized. Dietary supplement research and information expressed herein should be considered anecdotal in nature or opinions and hypotheses rather than generally accepted science. Unless otherwise noted, the studies presented herein may not have adhered to the strict regulatory controls required for approval of applied nutritional claims. Except where otherwise noted, some unpublished studies referenced herein have not been subjected to peer review in independent scientific journals. None of the information published herein may be used to suggest that any dietary supplement is a generally accepted treatment, preventative, cure or mitigation for any disease, except where approved as a permissible health claim pursuant to current regulation. See the FDA's Center for Food Safety and Applied Nutrition Website for more information about approved health claims for dietary supplements.

Limits of Liability and Disclaimer of Warranty

The author and publisher shall not be liable for your misuse of this material. This book is strictly for informational and educational purposes.

Warning – Disclaimer

The purpose of this book is to educate and entertain. The author and/or publisher do not guarantee that anyone following these techniques, suggestions, tips, ideas, or strategies will become successful. The author and/or publisher shall have neither liability nor responsibility to anyone with respect to any loss or damage caused, or alleged to be caused, directly or indirectly by the information contained in this book.

A Note From The Author

Together we can achieve so much more than individually. If, after reading this book, you want to learn more, make an appointment, book me for speaking engagements or join my team, please contact me directly. I have helped countless individuals look, feel and perform their very best, generate additional income and live the life they were meant to live.

Get Your Four Pillars To Healthy Living Checklist!

Use this valuable tool to keep you on the right path towards optimal cellular health!

With this checklist you'll be able to track your progress towards:

* Eating Healthy

* Training Functionally

* Activating Your Body's Cellular Pathways

* Healing From Within

Go to www.AnythingIsPossibleFitness.com to pick up your FREE checklist today.

www.AnythingIsPossibleFitness.com

Rick Binder

PO Box 22735

San Diego, CA 92192

(858) 707-5606

Rabinder2006@gmail.com

www.AnythingIsPossibleFitness.com

About the Author

Rick Binder is a Certified SCENAR Therapist and San Diego's leading Cellular Health Expert. His passion is health and wellness and his mission is helping and informing others on the direction of scientific and medical research pertaining to activating the body at the cellular level in order to eliminate pain, repair soft tissue injury and reduce oxidative stress – the root cause of hundreds of ailments and diseases. The end result is that his clients look, feel and perform at their optimal level.

He has led workshops and seminars for individuals and business leaders. He is involved with the local business and philanthropic communities, and he is a Board Member of the La Jolla Golden Triangle Rotary Club.

Rick earned his MBA in Global Management from the University of Phoenix in 2005. In addition he holds Certified Personal Trainer, Corrective Exercise Specialist and Senior Fitness Specialist designations from the National Academy of Sports Medicine

(NASM), he is a Certified TRX Instructor and he is TRX-Certified in Sports Medicine.

DR. ADAM - "BEING A PERSON OF SCIENCE..."

The Acupuncturist who had originally referred me to Rick showed me a video in relation to a healthcare supplement designed to reduce oxidative stress in the human body. I am well aware that oxidative stress causes inflammatory conditions that potentially lead to disease and dysfunction. I was a bit skeptical at first because my usual take on life is: "If something is too good to be true, it usually is." This product has been a life-changer in the affects that it has had on my overall well being.

Being a person of science who believes in investigational methods and evidence to support theory, I decided to write a 30-day journal using my first bottle. As a Chiropractor, I believe in fixing the issues that 'cause' dysfunction and lead to disease in the human body. I figured I would track the main 3 aspects of health: 1) Mental, 2) Physical, and 3) Chemical factors.

The main thing I noticed was how my mood changed, as well as my ability to heal. By day 9, I actually had an inversion injury of my right ankle. The usual swelling and throbbing pain characteristics were present. But by day 11, I was able to put weight on my ankle, and was able to have better mobility overall. It seemed unbelievable that in just 2 days I was able to move again after such a terrible injury. Less than a week out from the time of the injury I was able to be fully mobile again, and by 10 days out after the injury I was back to doing leg workouts.

The biggest change aside from the injury repair that I noticed has been the ability to better handle emotionally and mentally stressful situations. I am better able to have a clear, level-headed approach to figuring out how to best assess a situation and act upon it in an intelligent manner. If anyone would ask me about my experience and association with Rick I would simply tell them: "What are you waiting for?"

~ Adam McBride, DC

Dr. Adam McBride is originally from Lexington, MA, and he graduated from Syracuse University in 2008 with a Bachelor's Degree in Health and Exercise Science. He received his Doctorate Degree in Chiropractic from Life University in 2015. Dr. McBride utilizes a variety of techniques for proper treatment of his patients. He and has worked as a personal trainer and physical therapy assistant in the past. He specializes in rehabilitative methods such as Active Release Technique (ART) and corrective exercises for restoration of movement patterns contributing towards injuries.

CATHELIYA - "IF THIS STUFF REALLY WORKS, IT COULD..."

Ever since I can remember I have been suffering with extreme pain from my periods. When I hit the age of 28 the bleeding became heavier and heavier. I have been to multiple gynecologists, had all the tests run, did the ultrasounds and x-rays. They all told me everything was normal and that I was in perfect health! What a crock!!

By Age 40 it was out of control and I was sure one day I would die of this excessive bleeding. No one can bleed this much and survive. It was a heavy burden.

In 2015 I went to a new doctor. I told her the same things I told everyone else. By now though, she said I might be anemic and maybe fibroids would show up. I went to see the gynecologist and she said that my uterus was swollen. She said not to worry as this was an easy fix. She matter-of-factory said she would simply remove my uterus. I thought to myself "That easy for you to say!" but for me that wasn't an option. "I'm a holistic healer!!" I told her. "No one is taking anything out of me!!" As I was leaving she patted me on my shoulder and told me she had it done in her 30's and she was doing great. "How nice for you." I though to myself. The ultrasound revealed that I had several fibroids on my uterus and my blood work came back I was anemic.

I'm a massage therapist and a holistic healer, and I have been in the health and wellness industry for over 10 years. In between that I owned a caregiving service for over 4 years. I've seen quite a bit and I know a thing or two about illness and how it works.

I sat down with Rick and he introduced me to all that he was doing in regards to Cellular Health. He had me watch a short introductory video, and halfway through I thought to myself. "Wow!!!! If this stuff really works, it could solve my anemia, fibroids and the swollen uterus problems". I started taking the products. I had a few flare ups while taking it but I stuck to my belief that if it could help these other people it could help me.

My very next ultrasound they found only 1 tiny fibroid left, and is was so small they couldn't measure it. I am now on my way to recovery and back to slowly working out to get my health back into shape again.

I was also treated by Rick Binder a few times last year and started treatment again this year. His treatment is very effective. I have had tight neck and shoulder pain for most of my life. I have come to understand that I am a sensitive person, and I take on other people's stress on top of my own sometimes. My shoulders used to burn with pain in my 20's. Then the pain moved to my arms and pecs. The pecs were unbearable pain. I couldn't sleep or move well. I didn't have full range of motion without pain. Ricks treatments really helped a lot. I am sleeping with less pain and have better range of motion and no pain!

~ Catheliya Suwanakrit

Catheliya Suwanakrit is a Clinical Massage Therapist specializing in Massage Cupping, Craniosacral Therapy, Aroma Therapy, and Holistic Healing. She has been in the health and wellness industry for over 10 years.

MARILYN - "I AM A DIABETIC AND I HAD..."

I had Rick work on my feet and my neck, both of which have been huge issues and very painful for many years. I am a diabetic and have neuropathy on my feet. Since seeing Rick I have been symptom-free for some time now. I have had a few car accidents where my neck was severely damaged. It is significantly (70%) better. The treatment modalities that Rick uses are amazing and wonderful, and I would highly suggest it to anyone who's open to getting better.

~ *Marilyn Salerno*

Marilyn Salerno is a Certified Master Practitioner of Hypnotherapy and a graduate of the American Pacific College in Hawaii. She has certificates as a Practitioner of Hypnotherapy, Master Practitioner of Hypnotherapy, NLP, Time Line Therapy, Advanced Hypnotherapy and Clinical Hypnotherapy. Her classroom instruction was with Dr. Matthew B. James, M.A., PhD, Certified Master NLP trainer. She follows the Master Association for Integrative Psychology Training Standards guidelines.

DR. JOCELYN - "I HAVE SEEN GREAT PROGRESS..."

As a Doctor of Oriental Medicine I have a great deal of respect for medicinal herbs and formulas, especially because they are prepared for each individual and their particular circumstances. When Rick introduced me to his approach I was skeptical at first. His solutions were very different from any I had used before, but after experiencing them first-hand I can absolutely tell you that they work, as I have seen great progress in my own health and that of my patients. I will also continue to incorporate them into my practice from now on.

~ *Dr. Jocelyn Joy*

Dr. Jocelyn Joy, owner of Joy Acupuncture Health Centre is a Doctor of Acupuncture and Oriental Medicine. She has been successfully treating patients with chronic pain and illness for the past 15 years in

San Diego, Ca. She finds that Acupuncture and Herbal Medicine are the best tools she has at her disposal because they help spark the body's natural healing abilities and don't have side-effects.

JANINE'S STORY - "TRADITIONAL ANTI-INFLAMMATORY DRUGS DID NOTHING FOR ME"

I would like to share my experiences with Rick Binder and a few of his services that have improved my life and health.

In June of 2015 I was told I was missing a piece of cartilage from my left knee from a Physician in NY. I was told 3 shots of Euflexa would solve the pain issue and I would be fine for a while. I went ahead with this procedure but absolutely NO relief came from it.

In July I met Rick Binder and told him my story. Rick explained his Cellular Health philosophy of healing the body from the inside out and I figured "What do I have to lose?" I worked with Rick and followed his suggestions, and within a week I started to feel relief. I was able to go up and down stairs with little or no pain at first and it progressed to total relief. I was able to jump up from a kneeling position on a paddle board to a standing position without hesitation. I've been taking this supplement for 8 months and my knee pain is almost completely gone. Besides the pain, the inflammation I was feeling when kneeling has improved so much. I was unable to kneel on the left side. It felt stiff and very full inside. Rick treated my knee and – along with an all-natural supplement he introduced me to -

made a remarkable improvement. My knee was more flexible and the fullness I had been feeling improved tremendously.

I have an elbow injury from a few years ago that has been aggravated by recent overuse. Rick has been treating my elbow for a couple weeks and I'm seeing amazing improvement. My pain level has improved from about a 9 to a 3 almost overnight. It is an ongoing mission but I am seeing a definite decrease in pain and inflammation. The strength in my arm is improving and I am now able to lift items with that arm/elbow.

Traditional anti-inflammatory drugs did nothing for me. Joint specific injections that presented themselves as cures did nothing for me or my situation. Working with Rick has helped my quality of life by eliminating my pain and giving me my life back. I will be forever grateful to Rick for this.

If you are tired of taking medications that do nothing for you and that are potentially toxic to your insides then these natural non-invasive methods are definitely worth a look see. I am very happy I tried his methods.

~ Janine Prezzano

Contents

About the Author..ix

Introduction... 1

Part 1 What is Cellular Health?.................................... 11

Part 2 Old School Challenges......................................29

Part 3 The Four Pillars of Cellular Health.......................55

Pillar #1 Eat Healthy..59

The Future of Functional Nutrition is Now
by Nanci Tunley, NTC, FDN 67

Pillar #2 Train Functionally...71

Pillar #3 Activate Cellular Pathways.....................................79

Pillar #4 Heal from Within...87

Conclusion..99

Introduction

"The wind of change, whatever it is, blows most freely through an open mind."

~ Katharine Whitehorn

This book has been a long time coming. For a long time I wondered if it would ever get written at all. Bits and pieces of it have been bouncing around in my head for several years now and the events of my life over the past couple of years were both the final straws and missing pieces of the puzzle that, once experienced, finally gave me the conviction to sit down and get it done.

I've never really considered myself an author. In school it was all I could do to write a term paper. Even now my first drafts of this stuck pretty closely to *"The Elements of Style"* research paper format for citing sources. It was time-consuming and grueling, and I seriously considered shelving the entire project. Fortunately a good friend of mine - Donna Kozik (www.FreeBookPlanner.com) - set me straight, and from that point on the process became simple and the words seemed to flow.

Allow me to introduce myself. My name is Rick Binder, and I spent many years as a successful Executive Recruiter Los Angeles, where I ran the Consulting Operations for a very large international firm. My territory encompassed 6 offices throughout the Los Angeles, Ventura and Santa Barbara Counties. I was extremely good at my job and I was very well compensated for it.

When the economy imploded back in 2008 I found my position eliminated, and my role evolved into a more specialized role of finding jobs for healthcare finance executives for 1137 acute hospitals throughout the eastern seaboard. This was an incredibly eye-opening shift for me as I became immersed in the particulars of healthcare finance and what was truly important to the major players and executives. I'll give you a hint – it most certainly was NOT the patients well-being.

This was really the tipping point for me in terms of my recruiting career. I just didn't have the stomach for the level of hardcore nastiness required to advance any further into management in that field. Don't get me wrong. I had a reputation for ruthlessness in my own right. In fact I used to joke that in an industry filled with assholes, I could "out-asshole" just about anyone, but it turns out I was so very, very wrong. It boggles the mind how poorly people can treat other people. Life, I decided, was way too short to be that harsh and that miserable.

I am very passionate about helping people. I really did try to do this as a recruiter. Truth be told for a long time I believed I was doing just that, but in reality the industry and the job market are such that only a very small percentage of people can truly be helped.

I now consider myself incredibly blessed. I'm quite fortunate to have finally realized my true purpose in life and to be able to work in the field of wellness. I am finally in a position where I can help improve the lives of everyone with whom I come in contact.

I've been involved with fitness, athletics and martial arts my entire life so in 2008 when that cosmic sledge hammer came crashing down and obliterated nearly every single aspect of my life - I lost everything and just about everyone practically at once - I found myself in a very dark and dismal place. It was just about then that I remembered a saying I'd once heard: "Sometimes you must embrace the darkness before you can see the light." I'm not certain who is credited with it, but it helped carry me through those dark, dark days.

It took a few years to dig myself out of the anger, sadness, frustration and heartache before I finally decided to branch out on my own as a Certified Personal Trainer in San Diego, California. I went into this new chapter of my life with tremendous gusto, but I soon realized that nearly every third person I met in San Diego was a personal trainer. Out of necessity I needed to evolve further. Jump ahead a few years and my practice has morphed into a field I like to refer to as Cellular Health. I am a Cellular Health Expert.

Cellular Health – as I see it – is the practice of activating the body at the basic level - the body's primary building blocks - to look, feel and perform at optimal levels. As a Cellular Health Expert I have been able to eliminate pain and inflammation, speed in the recovery of soft tissue injuries and significantly reduce oxidative stress (cellular damage commonly seen as a root cause of aging and over 200 diseases). To put it as simply as possible, this is a good thing.

In my capacity as a Cellular Health Expert, I am unique in a metropolitan area that is highly concentrated with a myriad of health and wellness practitioners from the traditional to the insane.

My relocation to San Diego and my evolution from Executive Recruiter to Personal Trainer to Cellular Health Expert was quite a challenging and eye-opening experience. I realized there was further growth that needed to occur. I had been a corporate guy for my entire career. For the first time I realized just how little control employees truly have. Like a fish in a bowl, there are only so many choices.

There were many things I had taken for granted when I came to San Diego. I was now a business owner – an entrepreneur – in an industry in which I had no experience and a market where I knew no one. I no longer had my corporate healthcare benefits. I had no intention of spending $1600 per month for COBRA so I set out to find a policy of my own. I'd done this before without incident and didn't really think it would be much of a problem. Boy, was I ever wrong!

I consider myself to be quite healthy. As a Personal Trainer I have to be. I discovered, however, that in 2012 - in anticipation of ObamaCare - health insurers were denying coverage to virtually all individuals and self-employed business owners. I found myself without healthcare insurance for the first time in my life. I found it very difficult to accept that someone as healthy as I was could be blindly turned down by some nameless, faceless, out-of-shape beancounter in a back office somewhere.

One of the reasons I moved to San Diego was to start fresh. There were simply too many sad memories in Los Angeles and there was nothing keeping me there any longer. The other reason was to be closer to my parents, sister and nephew – the only people I knew in the area.

My father was getting up there in age and it made sense to be closer so that I could help out and spend more time with him. While this wasn't the easiest thing to do it turned out to be the right thing. He became quite ill shortly after my move, and after a year of rapidly deteriorating health he passed away in 2014.

The back-to-back gut punches of being denied insurance coverage and the slow passing of my father impacted me greatly, and these experiences cemented my belief that a re-education of the American people needs to happen. While this re-education needs to occur in several areas I'll limit the scope of this book to healthcare.

My father was a football player in his youth. He played in college in the days before facemasks were mandatory. He was 6'2" and a bit over 200 pounds. He never looked heavy. He taught me how to play catch, hit a baseball, fish, shoot, and do all sorts of "guy stuff", and he would tell me about all the mischief he'd gotten into while growing up in Texas back in the 1930s and 1940s. For most of his adult life he had a series of sedentary jobs and didn't really exercise much. And of course growing up in Texas he loved that down-home cooking. Chicken-fried steak and pecan pie were particular favorites of his.

High blood pressure and cholesterol run in the family and my father was no exception. He had prescriptions for these issues for many years. As he got older, however, it seemed that more and more issues would pop up. When he passed away in 2014 at the age of 88 he was on over 30 prescriptions. Some of these were simply to treat the side effects of some of the other prescriptions. All this was in addition to a pacemaker and so many stents in his heart that the doctors amusingly referred to it as "full metal jacket".

To be fair all the prescriptions and hardware did manage to prolong his life. Western medicine is not without merit in this regard. In fact, it seems that western medicine has just about perfected the art of keeping a heart beating. The sad fact is that often times this comes at a very high cost - financially and otherwise. I don't believe that as a patient my father was treated with the respect he deserved, and I don't believe that he died with the dignity to which he should have been accorded. There, of course, some compassionate people handling his care while he lingered in that hospital bed, but there were several – doctors and specialists mainly – who were just cold and in one case downright disrespectful. The latter, I am happy to say, met the ruthless side of me. It turns out when you stand up to these condescending jerks with authority (and vent your displeasure to that persons supervisors) they become much less cold. From that point on he became much more humane in dealings with my father.

All of this backstory brings me to the conceptualization of this book. My purpose in writing this is to open your mind to alternative methods for healing and for living the healthiest life possible. It is possible, but only if we go beyond what has been for far too long the conventional wisdom and conventional treatment modalities of Western Medicine.

I'm going to begin by explaining what I mean by Cellular Health. I know many people who would do a deep dive into all the science behind how our bodies and our cells work. I am going to cover it as simply as I possibly can without resorting to convoluted medical jargon.

Once we have a cursory understanding of just exactly what cellular health is and how our bodies work in this regard I will move on to address some of the challenges we currently face. Healthcare reform is a polarizing issue these days and I fear it will continue to be for the foreseeable future. As I see it what's standing in the way of cellular health for the masses is an outdated belief system and a whole bunch of tightly closed minds. There are simply too many conflicts of interest and too much money at stake to embrace a cheaper, more effective system.

Finally, we will cover what I refer to as the "Four Pillars of Cellular Health" and how embracing them can help set you on the path to peak cellular health so that you really do look, feel and perform at your optimal level. At the end of this book I will reference some of the clinical studies that have been and are continuing to be published in this area. Again, my hope is to create a new way of thinking and addressing our health issues. We have the technology to do just that. The science is there to support this idea. Those in the know are seeing the results for themselves. The question here is...

Will you be among them?

Part 1
What is Cellular Health?

"Your body's ability to heal is greater than anyone has permitted you to believe"

~ Unknown

SALLY'S STORY - IN HER OWN WORDS

I have not been kind to this body over the last 68 years. Too much abuse, too little exercise, poor nutrition, insomnia; to say nothing about destroying my cells through 25 years of cigarette smoking, alcohol intoxication and painkillers! Though I was once active, degenerative disk disease and osteoarthritis has taken its course, leaving me with increased immobility, low energy, weight gain, and yes, even autoimmune thyroid disease.

Experiencing frustration, I sought to see a Medicine Specialist in May of 2014. I had high hopes and I was desperate so I laid down the $10,000 they were charging. When the four-month program ended last October and I was happy to be 40 pounds lighter, but the weight didn't stay off and I gained most of it back in a year's time.

This past December I knew I must address my health and well-being from a different angle, which is how I met Rick Binder. Rick spent time getting to know my situation and me, and he put together a program to address my mobility issues and hopefully with the goal of loosing some weight as well.

There were challenges in exercising due to my immobility. Just completing a squat was near impossible due to pain in my left knee. Ongoing restriction and pain also were present in my low back and right shoulder. Rick, recognizing this condition, spoke to me about a cellular approach that made sense to me. He treated my left knee after a workout one afternoon. This single treatment proved invaluable to my mobility! I noticed almost immediately an increased range of motion and zero pain. I'm ecstatic for the elimination of pain, increased mobility and over 17 pound weight loss that has happened in just 6 weeks!

I found myself in the Emergency Room on January 1st with a kidney infection, and I had to limit my exercising for a few days. I actually thought I had a ruptured disk, because of the intolerable back pain I was experiencing at that moment. A follow-up with my primary care doc suggested the ongoing Degenerative disc disease, Bursitis of bilateral hips, the Sacroiliac joint, and of my right shoulder. She recommended a series of Steroid injections and Physical Therapy. I declined any Steroid injections and PT. My previous experience with these modalities had very little effect in the past. My treatment for these joint issues has been Tramadol and Meloxicam for the past 8 years, and previous to that mega doses of Ibuprofen. I'm usually controlled fairly well with the synergistic use of these Meds. They allow me to "move", and go about my day.

Rick worked on my back and hip as he had done before. I wasn't disappointed! I've had two treatments on my low back/hip, and though I know I need further treatment the results are quite remarkable! The outcome is liberating, I can bend and move with greater flexibility and agility! WOW! It's so exciting to walk effortlessly with a nice stride and a spring in my step!!!

A little over a month ago, Rick suggested introduced me to an all natural supplement that was supposed to lower Oxidative Stress in my body. We discussed the importance of cellular healing and how our bodies can repair themselves. It made sense but I was skeptical. I may not have been totally convinced but something is happening within my body. I have had terrible insomnia for years. I do not sleep soundly through the night. Recently, about

10 days ago, I noticed sleeping for six straight hours without interruption through the night. This is HUGE! I usually schedule all my appointments for mid-afternoon because I can't motivate/move in the morning. Well, next week Rick has me scheduled for a 9:30am appt. I've created a "motto" for myself; REPAIR, REGENERATE and REJUVENATE! This is absolutely MIRACULOUS!

I realize it's not too late to heal oneself through targeting and regenerating those cells of my body. Would I recommend Rick and the healing modalities that he offers? YES, in a heartbeat!

~ Sally Jacobus

SO WHAT IS CELLULAR HEALTH?

Someone once said, "Your body's ability to heal is greater than anyone has permitted you to believe." I believe this to be absolutely true. I believe this because we are seeing what the power of holistic wellness can do to heal ourselves. Acupuncture, massage and meditation have been around for thousands of years. To be fair so has surgery.

Each of these modalities - and others as well - have evolved over time to their present form, and they will no doubt continue to evolve. Science has evolved as well throughout this time. We know so much more than we did a thousand years ago, a hundred years ago, even a year ago. Cellular health wasn't even conceptualized until fairly recently, but I assure you this will be the apex of science and of healing in the near future. It's here now but the majority of the population has no idea what it is and are too closed minded to investigate. Suzy Kassem was quoted as saying *"The ego is what drives a self-serving individual who hates to admit they are wrong."* We must all check our egos at the door and open our minds to what is possible. Healing our bodies at the cellular level is possible because it is being done right here, right now.

Earlier I defined Cellular Health is the process of activating the body at the cellular level for the purpose of looking, feeling and performing at our optimal levels. Allow me to break this down so we are all on the same page.

Our bodies are composed of roughly 10 trillion (that's 10,000,000,000,000) individual cells. The largest of these cells is about the diameter of a human hair but most are much smaller than that. These cells are divided into approximately 200 different kinds of cells – liver cells, muscle cells, heart cells, skin cells… You get the idea.

Enzymes do the work inside of our cells. In a relatively basic type of cell – a bacteria such as E. Coli for example – there are roughly 1000 enzymes floating around at any given time. Most human cells are considerably more complex and thus have more.

These enzymes are basically where the chemical reactions occur in cells. In fact the purpose of enzymes is to allow cells to quickly carry out these chemical reactions. These reactions low the cells to build things or take things apart as needed, and it is how cells grow and reproduce.

Enzymes are proteins made from Amino Acids. They are formed by stringing together somewhere between 100 and 1000 amino acids in a very specific order. Simply put, proteins are any chain of among acids, and amino acids are the building blocks of Protein. The human body is approximately 20% protein by weight. Another 60% is water weight, and the remainder is composed of minerals such as calcium in the bones. There are around 100 amino acids available in nature, though it takes only 20 to construct the human body.

There are two basic types of amino acids – Essential and Non-Essential or Conditional. Essential amino acids also referred to as indispensable - are those you must get through the foods you eat. The human body can't make them. Of the 20 amino acids that compose a human being nine are essential, though adults only need eight of them: valine, isoleucine, leucine, lysine, methionine, phenylalanine, threonine and tryptophan. Histidine - the ninth amino acid - is only essential for infants. Since the body cannot store amino acids it must receive a regular daily supply which is why a healthy diet is of such importance in maximizing cellular health.

The body synthesizes non-essential and conditional amino acids are synthesized by the body. They aren't an essential part of our diet. Of the 11 non-essential amino acids, eight are considered conditional amino acids. Sickness and significant stress can make it so that the body may not be able to produce enough of these amino acids to meet its needs. Conditional amino acids include arginine, glutamine, tyrosine, cysteine, glycine, proline, serine and ornithine. The remaining three -- alanine, asparagine and aspartate -- are non-essential.

So long as the cell membrane is intact and manufacturing all the enzymes it needs to function properly the cell is alive. The enzymes allow the cells to reproduce, to create energy from glucose, to construct and maintain the cellular wall and produce new enzymes. The driving force behind all of this is in our DNA. Our DNA lies within our cells. It is a pattern of chromosomes and genes that in humans is approximately 3 billion blocks long.

HOW DOES THIS TIE INTO THE BIGGER PICTURE?

As you are no doubt beginning to understand, cells are the fundamental units of life. Cells constantly communicate with each other. When the body is in perfect balance, or homeostasis, it looks, feels and performs at optimal levels. Homeostasis is defined as the tendency of the body to seek and maintain a condition of balance or equilibrium within its internal environment, even when faced with external changes. Every function of the body communicates harmoniously in order to maintain a homeostatic state. Maintaining a body temperature of approximately 98.6 degrees would be an example of homeostasis. When something interferes with this - stress, injuries, pathogens, disease, etc. - it disrupts this harmonious communication.

Suffice to say that there is quite an amazing and complex infrastructure that goes into making a healthy human being. In order to remain as healthy as possible for as long as possible we want to make sure our cells remain healthy and free from damage. Cellular damage can result in the death of individual cells, mutations such as cancer, tissue damage, organ failure or even death of an entire organism.

What causes cellular damage? It turns out there are a great many things that damage our cells. Harmful molecules are constantly bombarding our cells – the air we breathe, the foods we eat, our lifestyle choices, etc. By now most everyone is familiar with the term "Free Radicals". Free radicals are atoms or groups of atoms with an odd number of electrons. They are formed when oxygen interacts with certain molecules. Another term we are becoming more familiar with is Oxidative Stress that is, simply put, a type of rusting from the inside out. An example of this rusting is when you cut an apple and leave it on the counter, and it starts to turn brown.

Once formed these highly reactive free radicals can start a chain reaction, like dominoes, and damage our cells. To prevent free radical damage the body has a defense system of antioxidants. Antioxidants protect our cells by absorbing these free radicals and counteracting the effects of oxidative stress.

Oxidative Stress is essentially an imbalance between the production of free radicals and the ability of the body to counteract or detoxify their harmful effects through neutralization by antioxidants. This is a term that has been around for quite some time. Currently there have been over 150,000 independent research studies on oxidative stress published in PubMed.gov. PubMed is a service of the US National Library of Medicine®. It provides free access to MEDLINE®, the NLM® database of indexed citations and abstracts to medical, nursing, dental, veterinary, health care, and preclinical sciences journal articles. It also includes additional selected life sciences journals not in MEDLINE. I've often heard it described as being akin to the Library of Congress for all independent medical and scientific research.

ANTIOXIDANTS

We have known about antioxidants for years now. Just about everyone can rattle off a list of several antioxidant-rich foods like blueberries, broccoli, red wine, dark chocolate, fronts and vegetables. In addition, antioxidants are commonly added to food products to prevent or delay their deterioration from oxidation.

Everywhere you look there is information on antioxidants. Now we've even coined terms like super-antioxidants and superfoods that everyone should be consuming in mass quantities to protect against these deadly free radicals. Moreover, pharmaceutical and vitamin companies are coming out with a slew of antioxidant supplements to really give those free radicals the knockout blow.

Antioxidants can be divided into two types – Direct (exogenous) Antioxidants and Indirect (endogenous) Antioxidants. We are mostly familiar with direct antioxidants that come in the form of food and supplements we take. They combat free radical damage to our cells, but how effective are they really?

Direct antioxidants originate from outside sources such as food, vitamins and liquids, and they counteract free radicals at a 1:1 ratio. That means for every direct antioxidant molecule we ingest we eliminate one free radical. This sounds like a fair enough trade off. The problem, however, is that with 10 trillion cells in the human body each generating multiple free radicals it's virtually impossible to consume enough direct antioxidants to make even a small dent. Imagine, if you will, a skyscraper that is completely engulfed in flames. Now imagine you're trying to put out this fire with a shot glass full of water. That's never going to work and eventually that building will be a smoldering pile of ash. THAT is roughly the equivalent of attempting to eliminate free radicals from our bodies by consuming direct antioxidants.

Indirect Antioxidants are those stemming from internal factors. We manufacture these from the inside. That's right. our bodies have the capability to make our own antioxidants when the proper internal pathways are activated from within. The more effective our bodies are at activating these pathways the better they are at offsetting harmful free radicals within our cells. To use the same example as in the previous paragraph, imagine putting out that building fire with a sprinkler system and a fire hose in each room in the midst of a heavy rainfall. That is the power of indirect antioxidants. Rather than the body neutralizing one free radical molecule for every antioxidant monoculture ingested, these indirect antioxidants neutralize free radicals at a rate estimated to be roughly 1,000,000 free radical molecules per second, every second. Given the choice I'm pretty certain most people would prefer the indirect route.

I'm not saying that we shouldn't eat a healthy diet rich in antioxidants – we most definitely should. It would appear, however, that perhaps our tried and true way of thinking might be just a bit out of date. Just how out of date? Well, we don't see many pay phones anymore, and I'm pretty certain dial-up internet is a thing of the past. Not to mention that with all the commotion about GMO's and heavily processed foods that remain apart of the standard American diet it just seems safer to have our bodies MAKE our own antioxidants from within.

NRF2 - A NEW REALITY

At this time I'd like to introduce to you the significant research and discoveries being made currently in the area of Nrf2. According to the website, Nrf2.com, *"Nrf2 is a powerful protein that is latent within* *each cell in the body, unable to move or operate until it is released by an **Nrf2** activator. Once released it migrates into the cell nucleus and bonds to the **DNA** at the location of the Antioxidant Response Element (ARE) or also called hARE (Human Antioxidant Response Element) which is the master regulator of the total antioxidant system that is available in ALL human cells."*

Did you catch that? The **MASTER REGULATOR OF THE TOTAL ANTIOXIDANT SYSTEM**. That, it turns out, is pretty HUGE.

It goes on to say that *"Activation of Nrf2 essentially opens the door for the production of a vast array of our body's most important antioxidants."* At this time PubMed.Gov lists over 6,100 published independent research studies pertaining to Nrf2 and this number is growing all the time.

Just how significant is the discovery of Nrf2 and its potential? In February of 2015 researchers at Washington State University published a study which states *"...we may be on the verge of a new literature on health effects of NRF2 which may well become the most extraordinary therapeutic and most extraordinary preventative breakthrough in the history of medicine."* In the HISTORY OF MEDICINE! Are you kidding me? How is this NOT front page news?

The study continues on and includes a table listing

several diseases where raising Nrf2 is reported to be useful in prevention and/or treatment in animal models and/or humans include:

Cardiovascular diseases

Neurodegenerative diseases such as Alzheimer's, Parkinson's, ALS and Huntington's

Cancer prevention

Chronic Kidney diseases

Metabolic diseases such as Type 2 Diabetes, metabolic syndrome and obesity

Certain types of toxic liver disease

Chronic lung diseases including emphysema, asthma and pulmonary fibrosis

Sepsis

Autoimmune diseases

Inflammatory bowel disease

HIV/AIDS

Multiple Sclerosis

Epilepsy

NUTRIGENOMICS

Nutrigenomics, also referred to as Nutritional Genomics, is the study of how foods affect our genes and how individual genetic differences can affect the way we respond to nutrients (and other naturally occurring compounds) in the foods we eat. It is essentially the combination of nutrition and genomics for the purpose of researching the various ways people respond to food based upon their individual genetic make-up. Human beings are very similar genetically but each of us have slight differences in our genetic blueprints that make us unique from everyone else. Think of it as a nutritional fingerprint. This nutritional uniqueness is a key determinant of the manner in which nutrients affect our bodies and in how we are able to metabolize the food we eat.

According to the Center of Excellence for Nutritional Genomics (CENG) at the University of California, Davis *"The promise of nutritional genomics is personalized medicine and health based upon an understanding of our nutritional needs, nutritional and health status, and our genotype. Nutrigenomics will also have impacts on society from medicine to agricultural and dietary practices to social and public policies and its applications are likely to exceed that of even the human genome project. Chronic diseases (and some types of cancer) may be preventable, or at least delayed, by balanced, sensible diets. Knowledge gained from comparing diet/gene interactions in different populations may provide information needed to address the larger problem of global malnutrition and disease."*

If the science continues to play out it offers up the very real possibility of personalized nutrition – a specific combination of nutrients capable of unlocking your optimal genetic balance. It all hinges on this two-way relationship between the nutrients we ingest and our genes. Imagine having a specific formula – one that has little or nothing at all to do with synthetic pharmaceuticals and their side effects – that can potentially prevent you from developing cancer, Alzheimer's, Multiple Sclerosis, Autism, Diabetes or even obesity! The possibilities are mind-boggling!

We are at the dawning of a new era. These are very real possibilities in our lifetimes. Some of this exists currently, and I truly believe it lies within these Four Pillars.

So, to summarize, we have approximately 10,000,000,000,000 cells in our bodies and each of these cells is constantly generating free radicals. These free radicals are harmful to our cells. Antioxidants offset these free radicals so we want to get them inside our bodies to fight the nasty free radicals.

There are two types of antioxidants. The kind we are most familiar with are direct antioxidants and we get them by eating antioxidant-rich foods and supplements. These direct antioxidants offset free radicals at a 1:1 ratio. On the other hand there are indirect antioxidants. These are the ones our bodies are capable of manufacturing internally and they offset free radicals at a 1:1,000,000 ratio. Indirect antioxidant production can be fired up by activating the Nrf2 pathway in our bodies.

This Nrf2 pathway has been (and continues to be) researched, and it is now considered to be the MASTER REGULATOR OF THE TOTAL ANTIOXIDANT SYSTEM! Scientists are publishing results of several independent, peer-reviewed studies of their findings with regards to Nrf2 and it has been referred to as "…THE GREATEST DISCOVERY IN THE HISTORY OF MEDICINE."

Are you still with me? Big pharmaceutical companies are aware of this research and they are busy chasing down synthetic ways of activating this pathway in our bodies. A few of them have actually succeeded and market these formulations as treatments for certain diseases. While this is certainly a step in the right direction these medications are wildly expensive and the list of potential side effects are horrifying to say the least.

This is an area that I believe has more potential to help a wider demographic in the supplement category. Supplements are not taken as seriously as prescription medications by regulatory agencies and the more traditional Western Healthcare industry but I really do believe they should be. But first we need to break down some very old-school thinking.

Part 2
Old School Challenges

"In a time of universal deceit, telling the truth is a revolutionary act."

~ George Orwell

Bud Fox: How much is enough, Gordon? When does it all end, huh? How many yachts can you water-ski behind? How much is enough, huh?

Gordon Gekko: It's not a question of enough, pal. It's a Zero Sum game – somebody wins, somebody loses. Money itself isn't lost or made, it's simply transferred – from one perception to another.

Bud Fox: How much is enough, Gordon?

Gordon Gekko: The richest one percent of this country owns half our country's wealth, five trillion dollars. One third of that comes from hard work, two thirds comes from inheritance, interest on interest accumulating to widows and idiot sons – and what I do, stock and real estate speculation. It's bullshit. You got ninety percent of the American public out there with little or no net worth. I create nothing. I own. We make the rules, pal. The news, war, peace, famine, upheaval, the price per paper clip. We pick that rabbit out of the hat while everybody sits out there wondering how the hell we did it.

~ From the Movie "Wall Street", 1987

OUR HEALTHCARE SYSTEM IS BROKEN

When I was originally thinking about a title for this book the first one to pop into my mind was "Why

Western Medicine Is Killing Us and What We Can Do About It". It's not that I was trying to be controversial or a fear-monger. I'd simply had enough of doctors with their condescending attitudes and certainties. I was tired of health insurance carriers who dole out their limited yet overpriced protection in an unjust manner that a team of nameless, faceless beancounters somewhere consider to be the most profitable to the executives and shareholders. I was frustrated with the unholy alliance between pharmaceutical companies and the FDA and just about everything they seem to stand for these days. Finally, I was sick to death of Congress for supporting all of this with seemingly no interest or concern for anyone but themselves. Perhaps I'd feel differently if I were privy to their guaranteed top-of-the-line healthcare for life.

I suddenly felt as though I had quite a bit to say about this topic. As the character Howard Beale in the 1976 movie "Network" so aptly shouted, *"I'm as mad as hell, and I'm not going to take this anymore!"* I was mad as hell too, and I decided then and there to do something about it.

Fortunately, I had the good sense to send my first draft to a very good friend and client of mine who talked me down off the ledge and explained that I'd connect more with my audience if it didn't sound like my own personal manifesto. After giving the matter more thought I made some changes and the project evolved into its present form.

That said I feel it's important to paint a picture of the current state of affairs. I do this not to vent my anger and frustration but to instead open people's minds into believing there just might be a better way. In so doing maybe on some small level the wings of change will take flight.

Healthcare in the United States, in my opinion, is backward. It's broken. Even the word "healthcare" is not an accurate description of what our system is at all. In order to call it healthcare the major players - hospitals, medical systems, doctors, insurance carriers, pharmaceutical companies and the FDA would have to actually care more about our health than they do about the almighty dollar. The sad fact is that in our current "healthcare" system profits trump people. We are not about curing disease at all. It's more about treating symptoms and covering risks of lawsuits.

PROACTIVE VS. REACTIVE

Imagine for a moment that you just bought a brand new car. It's shiny and clean and it drives like a dream. How do you feel driving it around town? Pretty great, right? The longer you drive it the more it ages. Potholes, traffic, the occasional fender bender, kids, spilled coffee, nicks and chips and scratches... How long do you think it will continue driving like a dream without proper maintenance? I'd be willing to bet that most of us couldn't imagine ignoring regularly scheduled maintenance on that shiny new car. Given the choice most of us would choose a proactive approach to regularly maintain our vehicle rather than the reactive choice of repairing the damage once it breaks down, right? Of course.

Now think for a moment about your body. Would you rather be proactive or reactive with your health? How many people do you know who don't exercise, eat poorly, smoke, drink to excess, ignore warning signs…? Suddenly it's no surprise as to why the obesity rate in the United States is roughly 70%.

We are a society that takes better care of our automobiles than we do our bodies. Don't believe me? Do you take your automobile in for its regularly scheduled maintenance? Oil changes? Tire rotations? Car washes and detailing? Tune-ups? Of course you do. Most of us wouldn't dream of buying a car and just driving it into the ground. To do so would be to shorten its useful life and lower its resale value. It's way cheaper to maintain our vehicles than it is to fix them once they break down, right?

What about our bodies? Wouldn't it also be less expensive to maintain them by eating the right foods in the right amounts, maintain our functionality, make sure our muscles are balanced and our structural integrity remains intact? Of course it would. Yet how many of us actually do this? Not that many really. If this were the norm then we wouldn't have an obesity problem in this country (or the world for that matter). I would go so far as to argue that many of the diseases and maladies that plague so many people would be far less prevalent.

THE PROBLEMS WITH WESTERN MEDICINE

Now let's look at our healthcare system. The problem with Western medicine is that it is completely reactive in nature. Think about this for a moment. How often do you go to a doctor aside from an annual physical exam – basically a blood test, a quick glance down the throat and in the ears, the always appreciated "turn your head and cough" and the ever pleasant "drop your pants and bend over the examination table" - for purely health maintenance? The answer is never because insurance won't cover it, doctors don't have the time for it and the general public doesn't make the time for it.

Western medicine is all about treating symptoms. Something doesn't feel right so we run to the doctor for a prescription, and all too often that prescription is in the form of an antibiotic or other pharmaceutical drug. The very idea of holistically healing the origin of the condition itself is virtually unheard of these days. This short-sighted and overly prevalent thinking doesn't focus on the root cause of what ails us. It doesn't heal the disease. In fact it often causes more harm to the patient through chemical medicines and invasive surgical procedures.

The trick is for us to adopt a proactive approach to healthcare as opposed to our current reactive approach. In order for this paradigm to shift on a societal level it will require education on a level our current government and healthcare systems seem to discourage. Our current system is simply too profitable for those in charge. Too many people have made their careers by limiting information and access and by "greasing the right wheels" to maintain this closely guarded cash cow that is our nations healthcare system. We MUST take a proactive approach to wellness or we will be forever at the mercy of our current healthcare system.

When I say proactive the reaction I usually get is "Rick, you mean I've got to join a gym and eat lettuce for every meal?" Proper nutrition and regular exercise are important of course. Really it's our current paradigms that are obsolete. By proactive I mean doing the things we know we must do in order to optimize our functionality and performance. A proper diet, exercise, rest and active recovery are of course a part of this, but there are other very simple steps we can take each day to make sure we look, feel and perform at our very best for as long as possible.

CONFLICT OF INTEREST

The way I see it there are several challenges facing us at this point. The root cause of just about all of them is really just one big conflict of interest. It's been present for a very long time and it's thoroughly ingrained into our very culture. There is a constant outcry for reform yet nothing really has improved.

Who's to blame here? Is it the FDA? Health Insurers?

Pharmaceutical Companies? Healthcare Providers? Congress? It's most likely a combination of all of the above for their overall closed-mindedness and for their focus on profits over people. Each of these topics could be the subject of a multi-volume expose in and of itself but for our purposes I'm only going to very briefly touch upon them.

FDA

The mission statement of the Food and Drug Association reads *"FDA is responsible for protecting the public health by assuring the safety, efficacy and security of human and veterinary drugs, biological products, medical devices, our nation's food supply, cosmetics, and products that emit radiation."* That sure sounds good, and to a large degree they do just that. It's actually rather frightening to imagine how bad things would be if there were no regulation at all.

First of all, does the FDA really have our best interests at heart? To some degree I'm sure they do, but how can we be certain? There are elected officials and other government higher-ups with ties to the food and drug industries who clearly have conflicts of interest. The FDA has gone on record in the past stating that *"Ultimately it is the food producer who is responsible for assuring safety"*. How can they, in good conscience, so flippantly pass the buck like this?

There are contradictory and confusing regulations regarding GMO testing and who's responsible for informing consumers. John Fagan, director of Earth Open Source and a noted expert in GMO testing, agrees. *"The big problem is that a voluntary non-GMO standard is diversionary,"* he says. *"It takes our attention away from the essential goal, which is to require labeling of all products that are genetically modified or that contain GMO ingredients or that are produced using GMO inputs or feed."* And let's not even get started on the fast food industry. Did you know that in the United States there are 19 ingredients in McDonalds French fries, yet in the UK there are only 3-4 ingredients in those same fries? Thank you FDA.

My point is that there are so many claims and instances of conflicts and cover-ups dating back over several years. Even if only a portion of it is true it's still true. Some of the more newsworthy FDA approvals include tobacco, GMOs, genetically modified salmon and certain food additives that are actually outlawed in other countries. The money at stake for a company to receive the FDAs approval is enormous. I'm just saying it calls into question just how impartial their rulings actually are.

PROFITS OVER PEOPLE

It seems as though we've lost our way in regards to healthcare in this country. Actually the problem goes way beyond healthcare but I'll do my best to stay on point here. My time as a healthcare finance recruiter gave me a great deal of insight into certain aspects of our health insurance and healthcare industries and I can tell you it's not about making Americans healthy. It is, but patients are secondary to profitability and the almighty dollar. If by denying a claim an insurance provider can save a couple bucks then so be it. People (i.e., future insured individuals) are being born every day so if they lose one today it's no big deal. Their coding system and methods for approving or denying claims make the US Tax Code seem like basic math. Physicians and healthcare systems must bill for multiple codes just to get one approved, and the patient is just a pawn in this very expensive and confusing game.

Healthcare Providers as well seem to have become more concerned with covering their own backsides than with the well-being of their patients. There are some good physicians out there who actually care but they are handcuffed in many ways by the healthcare system for which they work. Moreover, most doctors are very closed-minded and won't even acknowledge a holistic approach. Why? Because it's either not profitable or it opens them up to potential liability. There's not much money in treating patients who have no health issued requiring medication or surgery.

What if the healthcare system in America were to put people above profits? I'm not saying profits are bad. By the same token, those who provide medical treatment deserve to profit from their expertise. Certainly these companies need enough of a profit margin to recoup their operating costs and pay their salaries. I'm simply saying that people shouldn't go bankrupt paying for medical treatment.

It just seems to me there's a happy medium out there somewhere. Not that I'm a big fan of our banking system but they at least have usury laws in place. Rate caps would at least be a start. In lieu of that perhaps we should be able to know in advance the costs of the treatment we are about to receive. The Washington Post did a piece in 2015 about the "$153,000 Snakebite" that opens up, in my opinion, a whole big can of worms.

"In many cases, a hospital bill isn't actually a bill, but essentially an instrument in a complex negotiation between insurers and caregivers, with bewildered patients stuck in the middle. It's difficult to know which charges are real and which ones aren't, and which bills to pay and which ones to ignore. It's one reason medical debt is a huge factor in so many bankruptcies."

~ Washington Post, July 20, 2015

Why is it that everything else we purchase as a consumer has a specific price associated with it EXCEPT when it comes to seeing a physician? Sure, we know how much our co-pay will be – in some cases before the receptionist even greets you – but beyond that it's anyone's guess. Is there anything else besides our healthcare where we blindly purchase something without even a remote idea as to the cost? Of course not! That's ludicrous!

If those medical bills are simply negotiating tactics then why is that? What are they hiding from me? Shouldn't I be allowed to decide what tests and procedures cost BEFORE I purchase them? OF COURSE I SHOULD! Why do we allow this to go on? What can we do to put an end to this?

How can we sway the odds of receiving proper and compassionate care within the confines of our existing system that values profits over people? The answer lies in natural healing and in activating our bodies to maintain and heal ourselves from the inside out at the cellular level. In short, the answer lies in the Four Pillars of Cellular Health.

SURGERY VS. HOLISTIC

According to Webster's Dictionary, the term "surgery" is defined as *"Medical treatment in which a doctor cuts into someone's body in order to repair or remove damaged or diseased parts."*. Other reference sources define it as the branch of medicine that employs operations in the treatment of disease or injury. They go on to say that surgery can involve cutting, abrading, suturing, or otherwise physically changing body tissues and organs.

Holistic, on the other hand, is defined as *"relating to or concerned with whole or with complete systems rather than with the analysis of, treatment of, or dissection into parts. Holistic medicine attempts to treat both the mind and the body."* It is also suggested that each individual part of a whole person is intimately interconnected and explicable only by reference to the whole. Holistic medicine is the treatment of the whole person, taking into account mental and social factors, rather than just the physical symptoms of a disease. The very definition hints that there may be other, less invasive, less costly and less risky than what our typical Western Physicians – or more accurately the health insurance carriers – deem "medically necessary".

I'm not saying that surgery is bad or that there aren't times when surgical procedures are absolutely necessary. Of course there are. I'm simply saying that unnecessary surgery is bad. As previously stated there are times when surgery is necessary. In those instances surgery really does become the only viable choice in order to fix what's wrong. Pharmaceutical drugs have their place as well.

I'm simply suggesting that there are occasions where non-surgical alternatives are a very viable option. If a torn Rotator Cuff or a torn Meniscus, for example, were able to be repaired without the pain, invasiveness, risks of complications and infections, downtime, rehabilitation and recovery then wouldn't it be prudent to at least EXPLORE that option? Of course it would. And until such times as our healthcare system and the medical community comes around to this new reality it is up to us as consumers to seek out and be open to such options, provided of course that there is research to back it up.

OLD SCHOOL THINKING

The main problem we have as a society is that we've been conditioned for so long now that doctors know everything about everything and we don't question diagnoses, prescriptions, courses or treatment... On the contrary, we simply accept it as a matter of course.

We have been conditioned to respect doctors and even to revere them. How did this system come to be? That part is easy to answer – doctors themselves, and insurance companies, and the FDA. It doesn't help when mainstream television has dozens of hospital and doctor shows airing constantly, and in each case the doctors are portrayed as people who care about their patients to the exclusion of all else in this world. While I'm sure there are some doctors out there who truly do care that much, I'm quite confident that only a very small percentage of them can be found in the United States of America.

Just recently I was once again made aware of this fact. I had injured my wrist and for months it wasn't getting any better. The root problem was a pinched or bruised nerve and the pain was excruciating. I had been attempting the holistic route – Chiropractic, Acupuncture, Orthopedic Massage, SCENAR – and nothing even made a dent. Finally, I acquiesced and tried to get in to see a physician.

I must preface this by saying up to this point my holistic practitioners had managed to accommodate me and my total out-of-pocket expense had been about

$25 total. With each practitioner there was genuine empathy displayed. They squeezed me in and told me not to worry. At no point did I develop anxiety about the treatment or, more importantly, the cost, and I will say at the conclusion of my treatments there was some relief.

Now enter the Physician. The FIRST time I went in to see him (a specific Orthopedic Doctor) he wasn't in. His office would have had me see someone but if I needed a Cortisone injection as I expected then I would have to come back in two days when the Doctor was in the office. I returned two days later for the SECOND time at 1:30 in the afternoon only to be told that the Doctor wouldn't see me because he was leaving in a few minutes to attend a football game. I explained my situation and told them how painful this was and asked if he could just stick around for a few minutes. "No exceptions" was the answer I received from the stone-faced front desk attendant. Finally, two days later I returned (though I'm really not sure why) and on the THIRD visit I paid my $40 co-pay plus another $30 for a brace and was told to give it two weeks to see if it improved.

Jumping ahead a bit, it ended up being two more visits (at $40 co-pay per visit) before I was referred to a specialist. The specialist couldn't see me for a few weeks which pushed it into the new year. My NEW co-pay was now $55, and it took two of those visits plus another "special" brace which cost $50 to fix the problem.

At this point I'm still waiting to see what the remainder of the damage will be after the Doctor and the Insurance company finish their DMR Code dance. It's the unknown expenses that really do terrify me more than any medical procedure I may have to go through.

Perhaps I am stereotyping but that doesn't mean I am wrong. I recently was invited to speak at large active living community. During my presentation I took a straw poll to see who among the audience of 65-85 year olds were truly happy with their physicians and their responses genuinely surprised me. In this particular audience there was only one person who fell into this category. The overwhelming majority felt their doctors ranged from impersonal and distant to downright condescending. They believed them to be more concerned with peddling prescriptions and managing their own liability for doing so than they were about their patients. To be fair that's not exactly a peer-reviewed study of scientific significance, but it is interesting.

According to USA Today, *"...unnecessary surgeries might account for 10% to 20% of all operations in some specialties, including a wide range of cardiac procedures — not only stents, but also angioplasty and pacemaker implants — as well as many spinal surgeries. Knee replacements, hysterectomies, and cesarean sections are among the other surgical*

procedures performed more often than needed...".
I would argue that some of these procedures – especially those involving soft tissue injuries, could be repaired non-surgically with significantly reduced risks, recovery time or pharmaceuticals. I've helped people with knee, shoulder, ankle, neck and back injuries to reduce or eliminate pain and get back to their normal routines by simply activating their bodies at the cellular levels so that their bodies heal themselves. Sometimes this is a stand-alone treatment but it is also incredibly effective when done in conjunction with Chiropractic, Acupuncture, Physical Therapy or Massage as it effectively "locks in" that treatment and speeds up the healing process. I'll get into this in more detail shortly.

PHARMACEUTICAL COMPANIES

Pharmaceutical Companies, to be fair, do a lot of good. Without their expertise, research and hard work many of us would be much worse off from a health standpoint. That said, the extravagance and waste that goes on within the industry is a big part of why we have some of the most expensive and least effective healthcare in the civilized world.

Would it surprise anyone to know that in 2015 Pharmaceutical companies spent nearly $180,000,000 on lobbyists in the hope of influencing congress and government agencies?

According to an Alliance for Natural Health article, *"...the 'Catch-22' of drug economics—that no one will spend the exorbitant sums needed to run clinical trials if the product can't be patented and turned into a huge money-maker—practically ensures that natural prevention or treatment will be ignored."* I suppose I can't completely fault the pharmaceutical companies for this. After all, there are some incredibly rare diseases out there where the population of affected patients just wouldn't justify the tens of millions of dollars it might take to find a suitable cure.

Let's forget about the overwhelming majority of our population dependent upon prescription medications for the time being and simply focus on antibiotics.

ANTIBIOTICS ARE BEING OVERPRESCRIBED

Antibiotics are medicines used to treat infections or diseases caused by bacteria. They are used for a wide range of other infections caused by bacteria, including urinary tract infections, skin infections and infected wounds.

To be fair, antibiotics have saved millions of lives since they were first introduced in the 1940s and 1950s. It is their rampant and indiscriminate overuse that has created the problems we are seeing today. It is quite unfortunate that many antibiotics are no longer effective against the bacteria they once killed.

Clostridium difficile colitis, commonly known as C Difficile or C-Diff, is an infection of the colon by bacterium. Toxins are produced in the lining of the colon that damages the affected area and causes fever, diarrhea and abdominal pain. If left untreated, serious complications can occur which include dehydration, rupture of the colon, and the spreading of the infection to the abdominal cavity or body. In severe cases this can be life-threatening.

The most common cause of C-Diff is treatment with antibiotics as it is believed to suppress normal the colonic bacteria that usually keep C-Diff from multiplying and causing colitis.

Most cases of C-Diff colitis occur in patients in the hospital, but the number of cases that occur among individuals not in the hospital has increased greatly, in large part due to the widespread use of antibiotic treatments prescribed by physicians.

Here are some horrifying statistics according to the CDC:

# of C-Diff cases Annually	500,000
Excess health care cost (Acute care facilities only)	$4.8 Billion
Patients receiving antibiotics during hospital stay	More than 50%
Unnecessary hospital antibiotic treatments	30%-50%

That just seems to be an awful lot of unnecessary antibiotics. I'm not saying physicians should be 100% correct 100% of the time but that's WAY BEYOND what we should expect from our healthcare system.

Not finishing an entire course of antibiotic treatment can have some bad outcomes. Although you may feel better before your prescription is finished, it is possible that all the bacteria causing the infection have not been killed. This makes it more likely that the infection will not be cured and will quickly return once you stop taking the antibiotic. It can also increases the likelihood that the bacteria will become resistant to the antibiotic, and the next time you take the antibiotic it might not work as well.

THE GUT/BRAIN CONNECTION

Our digestive tracts have literally trillions of microbes or "gut flora". It has been estimated that approximately 15% of a person's total body weight can be attributed to these microbes. A healthy digestive tract should have a balance of roughly 85% good microbes to 15% bad microbes. In a perfect world this would be the case, but as we factor in external factors – the air we breathe, the processed foods we eat, our increasingly sedentary lifestyles and stress this ratio begins to change. The bad microbes begin to overtake the good ones, which ultimately weakens the body and the immune system.

Pathogens enter the body as the immune system begins

to break down, and the beginnings of sickness and disease start to form. As symptoms begin to surface we may end up running to a doctor. The doctor will make us feel better with their magic prescription pad, and in 10 minutes we are out the door with a fresh dose of antibiotics.

Antibiotics have the effect of killing off ALL of these microbes – both the good and the bad. The devastation this causes is akin to strip mining. It literally leaves the gut depleted of good microbes that regulate immune response regulating gut flora. This is very dangerous for our entire immune system, which may never fully recover.

We have become so accustomed to our frantic pace processed foods and feelings of general anxiety and unease that we are essentially blind to what's happening inside our bodies. Over and above the generalized Oxidative Stress damaging all of our cells is the chronic inflammation in our gut that—left unchecked—disrupts the normal functioning of many bodily systems.

Research is confirming more and more that there is a definite connection between our brains and our gut. Hidden in the walls of the digestive system is what scientists are now calling the Enteric Nervous System or ENS. It is comprised of two thin layers lining entire gastrointestinal tract from the esophagus all the way to the rectum, and it is comprised of more than 100 million nerve cells. Wrap your minds around this: this network of neurons in the gut is as vast and complex as the network of neurons in our spinal cord!

According to Doctor Jay Pasricha, M.D., director of the Johns Hopkins Center for Neurogastroenterology, *"The ENS may trigger big emotional shifts experienced by people coping with irritable bowel syndrome (IBS) and functional bowel problems such as constipation, diarrhea, bloating, pain and stomach upset. For decades, researchers and doctors thought that anxiety and depression contributed to these problems. But our studies and others show that it may also be the other way around. Researchers are finding evidence that irritation in the gastrointestinal system may send signals to the central nervous system (CNS) that trigger mood changes."*

So how can we repair the damage that's already been done? How can we affect the gut and the immune system?

1. The most immediate effects have been discovered simply by changing the way we eat. People who eat the most processed and highly refined foods seem to have a different gut composition than those who eat more whole foods, fruits and vegetables.

2. Though research is still in he early stages it does seem as though probiotics may help. Certainly they help repair some of the damage caused by antibiotics. Some things to be aware of here are:

a. Certain strains of probiotics (Lactobacillus and Bifidobacterium) have been found to be more effective than others in restoring the healthy "good" microbes in the gut and

b.   They are really only effective if they get to their intended destination (our intestinal tracts) alive – without being killed off and broken down by stomach acids.

Probiotic-rich foods include Yogurt, Kefir, Sauerkraut, Dark Chocolate, Microalgae, Miso Soup, Tempeh, Pickles, Kimchi and Kombucha. There are others as well, but it is important to note that not all probiotics are created equal.

For example, yogurt is widely known as having probiotic qualities. In reality, for yogurt to actually be yogurt by definition, it must have two strains of bacteria—Lactobacillus bulgaricus and Streptococcus thermophilus. The trouble here is that these strains are destroyed by the acidity of the stomach and the enzymes of the pancreas, so nothing reaches the colon and it's not beneficial. Some yogurts are now enriched with other live bacteria of different strains that do survive to their intended destination in the intestinal tract.

My point is that it can be difficult for the general public to know the difference so it's important to do your homework if you are eating specific foods for their perceived probiotic benefits.

ARE WE REALLY GETTING THE BEST MEDICINES?

According to the Center for Disease Control *"… prescription narcotic pain reliever overdose deaths now exceed the number of deaths from heroin and cocaine combined."* Can we really be sure our doctors are prescribing us the right drugs for the right reasons? Why do pharmaceutical companies feel the need to advertise their products to the general public? And why in these ads are we told to "ask your doctor or pharmacist"? First of all, pharmacists cannot prescribe these medications. Second, with prescription costs already out of control, why are pharmaceutical companies spending so many millions of dollars to advertise their drugs to such a mass audience when only doctors are allowed to prescribe them? I would think by not spending those hundreds of millions of dollars on media advertising that at least some of those savings could be passed along to the consumer.

Nearly 7 out of every 10 American adults are currently taking supplements for one reason or another. It begs the question, are they safe? The Alliance for Natural Health International, based in the UK, recently revealed data showing that adverse reactions to pharmaceutical drugs are 62,000 times more likely to kill you than food supplements and 7,750 times more likely to kill you than herbal remedies.

The data, which was collected from official sources in the UK and EU, demonstrate that both food supplements and herbal remedies are in the 'super-safe' category of individual risk – meaning risk of death from their consumption is less than 1 in 10 million.

Again, as concerned citizens and ambassadors of our own personal health and wellbeing we need to be aware of all this and take the necessary steps to protect ourselves. How do we do this? First of all open your mind. Learn about your options. This is America so you're always free to say "No", but if you're too short-sighted to learn something new then that's just plain ignorance. In short…

KNOW WHAT YOU'RE SAYING "NO" TO.

Do some research. Ask questions. Find out your options. If you are being prescribed antibiotics make sure it's necessary. Ask what you can do to replace and replenish your healthy gut flora. Seek out holistic options – but make sure those options are based in science.

Part 3
The Four Pillars
of Cellular Health

"You never change things by fighting the existing reality. To change something, build a new model that makes the existing model obsolete."

~ R. Buckminster Fuller

R. Buckminster "Bucky" Fuller was an American architect, systems theorist, designer, inventor and author who published more than 30 books. He developed numerous inventions, mainly architectural designs, and popularized the now widely known geodesic dome. He once said "You never change things by fighting the existing reality. To change something, build a new model that makes the existing model obsolete." I'm here to tell you that the existing model for healthcare in this country is obsolete. A new model is being developed, and more and more people are coming to this realization every single day. They are tired of rising costs, reduced services, increased risks and being treated like they don't matter. They want proactive WellCare. They want holistic options. They want knowledgeable service providers who actually care. They want natural remedies without side effects and synthetic ingredients.

We have now thoroughly covered the issue of Cellular Health. It's time now to elaborate and explain how this new model can help us to develop and maintain the healthiest cells possible. Some of this might sound familiar to you and it should be. The concepts have been around for years, yet there is so much conflicting information out in cyberspace that it's a challenge to know which way to turn.

The final two pillars, however, are new. I won't say they are controversial. The science is there. Let's just say they are not well known mainly because the mainstream media hasn't yet jumped on the bandwagon in their usual over-the-top fashion, and the medical community – as we've seen – isn't exactly willing to entertain anything new at this juncture. The time is rapidly approaching though.

So what are the four pillars? First, eat healthy. Second, train functionally. Third, activate cellular pathways. Fourth, heal from within. Let's spend the remainder of this book discussing each in more detail.

Pillar #1
Eat Healthy

"Let food be thy medicine and medicine be thy food."

~ Hippocrates

PRESCRIPTION VS. NUTRITION

First off, let me say that not all prescription drugs are bad. Conversely—and to be completely fair—not all supplements are good. I believe by taking a more proactive approach, such as avoiding processed foods, soda and tobacco, eliminating consumption of sugar and alcohol, monitoring caloric intake and drinking plenty of water, a person can significantly lower the risk of contracting certain diseases.

There is really nothing I can say here that we have not already heard, and no matter what side I lean towards there will be many opposing points of view. With so many fads, trends, "magic pills", workout regimens and reality weight-loss shows it's no wonder why there's so much confusion out there. Personally, I've found that most people can get behind a new way of eating as long as it's introduced properly with realistic expectations. I'm hoping I can at least add my two cents and dispel some of the myths and misinformation out there so that you can get back on that road to cellular health from a nutritional standpoint.

I introduced the term "Nutrigenomics" in an earlier chapter. Again, nutrigenomics is the study of how foods affect our genes and how individual genetic differences can affect the way we respond to nutrients (and other naturally occurring compounds) in the foods we eat. If, as this area of research continues to evolve, we actually crack the code and are able to design nutrition plans specifically suited to an individual's unique requirements then the endless volumes of contradictory diets, trends, opinions and assorted other trial-and-error nutritional protocols will become as obsolete as dial-up internet.

Optimizing cellular nutrition means giving your body the full range of vitamin and mineral requirements it needs - 19 micronutrients in all, including vitamins A, C, D, E, and K, plus the B vitamins, calcium, iron, magnesium, zinc, selenium and iodine - to offset the tremendous amount of oxidative stress and cellular damage which occurs on a continual basis. From a purely caloric standpoint this is nearly impossible to do. Remember, the antioxidants we consume through our diet are Direct Antioxidants which only offset one free radical per antioxidant molecule. Since our bodies are producing trillions of free radicals per day it's just not possible without the proper supplementation and resulting activation of our bodies antioxidant regulator pathways. That said, we still want to be eating in a manner that most efficiently addresses this issue.

How do we know how much of these nutrients are "adequate" to keep us healthy? For many years – actually since World War II – we have relied on the governments Recommended Daily Allowance (RDA), or Reference Daily Intake (RDI). That may have been fine back then but the world was a different place back then. There were less pollution and processed foods back then. Our lifestyles were much simpler and our stressors were far less severe than they are today, and while they were generally effective at lessening some of the big issues of the day back then – Scurvy, rickets… - they fail to account for many of the chronic degenerative diseases we face in our modern day culture.

Nutritional needs have evolved over the past 70 years and we need to change with the times. There is a great deal riding on proper nutrition. Namely less disease, stronger immune systems, better health and more productivity and functionality to name a few.

Optimal nutrition is not the same as following the RDAs. It is the level of nutrition required to prevent chronic degenerative diseases such as arthritis, Cancer, Alzheimer's, Osteoporosis, Diabetes and heart disease. Sadly, many doctors still believe in the RDAs as the baseline for optimal nutritional health. This antiquated belief combined with a general bias against nutritional supplements only serves to compound the problem.

So what can we do about this? How can we feed our bodies and give our cells the nutrients, vitamins and minerals they need when 1) we are following antiquated nutritional standards and 2) it is all but impossible to consume what our bodies need with food alone?

WHAT IS GOOD NUTRITION?

I am going to avoid making too many specific recommendations. Rather I'm offering up some rough guidelines. There are specific dietary restrictions and eating plans based on so many factors – Cancer Diets, Diabetes Diets, Weight-Loss Diets, Muscle-Building Diets, Healthy Gut Diets, Immune Booster Diets, Gluten-Free Diets... The list goes on. There are just so many variables it would be irresponsible to give a "one-size-fits-all" strategy.

1.   Avoid processed foods. I realize this can be a challenge given our busy lifestyles but it's wise to avoid heavily processed foods.

2.   As a general rule, try to stick to a diet where daily caloric intake is roughly 50% carbohydrates, 30% fat (two-thirds of this should be healthy unsaturated fats present in nuts, oils, fish, eggs, and avocados) and 20% protein. This can be modified accordingly based upon specific fitness, weight loss, muscle-building or specific health issues but the 50/30/20 plan is at least a place to start.

3.   Avoid added sugar. Added sugar is the single worst ingredient in the modern diet. According to the Center for Disease Control most Americans consume upwards of 16% of their daily calories in the form of added sugars. That is way above what we should be consuming. I'm not referring to natural sugars found in foods such as fruits and vegetables. Natural sugars actually do contain micronutrients as well as water and fiber. It is the added sugars we should be avoiding. The most common added sugars are regular table sugar (sucrose) or high fructose corn syrup, both of which

provide empty calories with no added nutrients and can damage metabolism in the long run.

4.   Limit sodium intake. The American Heart Association recommends keeping daily sodium intake to no more than 1,500 milligrams (about 1 ½ teaspoons). Most Americans consume more than twice that amount on a daily basis. The problem lies in processed and restaurant foods which are heavily laden with sodium among other ingredients we don't need to be consuming.

5.   Calories most certainly matter in terms of gaining, losing or maintaining weight, but not all calories are created equal. Also important are the actual foods we eat. Different types of foods have different effects on those feelings of satiety as well as ones hormonal levels and their overall health. Fructose, for example, is much more of an appetite stimulator than is glucose. Also, while protein can suppress appetite while also increasing metabolic rate when compared to the same amount of calories from carbohydrates or fat it can also help to repair and rebuild lean muscle mass which in turn burns more calories.

6.   Wheat, while often considered a more healthy option, is now seen as a contributor to various health issues. Wheat is largest source of gluten in our diets, and several studies are beginning to show increased sensitivity to it among a fairly significant percentage of the population. Gluten has been linked to contribute to symptoms such as digestive issues, stool

inconsistency, fatigue, pain and bloating. In addition it can damage the lining of the intestine in certain instances. Wheat gluten has even been associated with certain brain disorders including schizophrenia, autism and cerebellar ataxia in some controlled trials. The bottom line is that wheat is not nearly as healthy as we originally believed it to be.

At this point I'm going to pass the proverbial baton for a few moments. As I mentioned at the beginning of this segment I am not a nutritionist. I do offer nutritional counseling and in that regard I believe I do a pretty good job. My clients' results can attest to this fact.

That said, I enlisted the help of my friend Nanci Tunley, a Functional Nutritionist in the San Diego area. I think very highly of Nanci, and I have come to realize that she really knows her stuff. Since we share many of the same beliefs about food I thought I would let her contribute a portion of her vast wisdom here.

The Future of
Functional Nutrition is Now

by Nanci Tunley, NTC, FDN

The functional nutrition approach is at the cutting edge of health and healing. Going beyond the outdated "eat this for that" paradigm in traditional nutrition, functional nutrition seeks to restored balance and build health at the cellular level.

Ask 100 different nutrition professionals for an ideal diet is and you will receive one hundred different answers. Even in holistic and functional nutrition sectors there are many variations. Are they all right? Yes, but not for every body. Most consumers are completely bombarded and confused with marketing messages and conflicting studies. This leaves most people completely perplexed on how to proceed with a nutritious diet and worse, sometimes leads them to the wrong diet. So how do you know what you are doing is correct?

Ideally, to choose the best nutrient dense diet for your body from a functional perspective, you must have these three things:

1. A general knowledge of how the major systems in your body are functioning. This can be determined in many ways from lab work, questionnaire or physically depending on the modality of the practitioner. The hormonal, detoxification, immune, cardiovascular and digestive systems need to be considered among others. Any functional health practitioner can help with this.

2. A healthy relationship with your food and your body. Having a healthy relationship to your body allows you to tune into what foods work best for you as well as know when you are hungry and full. This is a simple, yet often missing piece for many people. The body will let you know what works for you and what doesn't. Learning to listen to your body's unique language is a crucial part of any eating plan.

3. A consideration of your unique genetics. Genetic testing can determine personal limitations or nutritional requirements some individuals require for optimal health. This is more important when the above efforts are being taken and improvement is not being seen.

No matter what diet you are eating the following suggestions are true for everyone:

Buy and consume whole foods as much as possible – eat REAL food. That means avoiding food from bags, boxes and cans. Items that contain added sugar, preservatives, trans-fats and artificial ingredients lack nutrition. In simpler terms, stay away from selections that have very long ingredient lists. Typically, once food labels begin to exceed five ingredients, they start becoming more of a risk to your health.

Avoid Most Diet Meal Plans. Sorry to say, but many of these commercial "diet meal plans" as advertised by a variety of celebrities are not healthy. All it takes is one look at the ingredient labels on such products to understand why they're dangerous – avoid them!

Cook your own food. Learn to prepare delicious meals that are healthy and help you reach your goals. If you don't feel like you have time to cook, adjust your schedule to make time. You can do almost a week's worth of cooking in one afternoon and freeze or refrigerate it.

Eat what is right for you. To fuel us properly, food must be of the purest form, of the right amount and tailored to your own genetic potential. This is also why most trendy diets today don't work for everybody. Listen to your body, and eat what makes you feel the best. If a food makes you bloated and tired, don't eat it! Eat what makes you feel energized and satisfied.

Maintain good glycemic control. Fluctuating blood sugar causes a great deal of stress on your body creating unpleasant symptoms, energy problems, and states of disease. Sugary foods can cause this fluctuation in blood sugar.

Document your progress. Perhaps the greatest tool you have is the ability to try something new and take note of any changes, for better or worse. Any climb back to health requires you to listen to your body, notice what is going on, and adjust according to what works.

In health + happiness,

Nanci Tunley, NTC, FDN

Nanci Tunley is a heart centered health transformation specialist. She blends cutting edge functional nutrition with heart centered coaching. She looks for the root cause to restore balance both physically and emotionally.

She specializes in suboptimal diet, blood sugar balance, hormonal imbalance, micronutrient deficiency, digestive disorders and detoxification. She often incorporates functional lab work into her programs to truly provide a bio-individual experience.

Pillar #2
Train Functionally

"Take care of your body. It's the only place you have to live."

~ Jim Rohn

BARB – "EXERCISE HAS BECOME A HABIT"

Rick has been my trainer for almost a year and he is the best. He understood my goals, needs and concerns (some injuries and physical concerns) and created a varied and appropriate program for me that targeted the way I move normally throughout my day. He checks in frequently to be sure I'm on track, and is always available to answer questions, tweak my exercises, draw pictures and, of course, tell jokes. He helped me make exercise a habit (rather than an irritation) and helped me become a more independent exerciser. I highly recommend him.

~ Barb, San Diego

GENETIC POTENTIAL

The area most often overlooked when it comes to exercise and our beauty-obsessed culture is genetic potential. At the peak of my martial arts training days - when I was as limber and strong and functional as I could be - my genetic makeup wouldn't allow me to do certain things. I would love to throw those beautiful kicks with one foot on the ground and the other straight up in the 12:00 position but I just don't have the flexibility.

Regardless of the training methods I use - even if I were to train and stretch and work on my flexibility 10 hours daily - I will never be able to do that. My body just wasn't designed to do certain things.

There are trainers, coaches and even parents who have

their clients and children follow dangerous training and nutritional programs in an attempt to maximize performance. That's not to say performance cannot be improved upon. I'm just saying that setting realistic goals and incorporating the most effective training methods available combined with lots of hard work and dedication is the key to maximizing our personal genetic performance.

FUNCTIONAL TRAINING

Traditional training at most bid gym chains have long revolved around machines and free weights. Next time you find yourself in one of these establishments take a few minutes to look around. You'll see most everyone there (at least those not admiring themselves in the mirrors, talking on their cellphones or texting their friends) either sitting down on a machine or weight bench or lying down on a machine or weight bench. Done correctly functional training is not about sitting down on a machine or lying down on a machine. It's entirely about BEING the machine.

My journey through the fitness profession has been a bit more roundabout than most. For many years it was just what I did out of pure enjoyment, but as I think back I've always stuck to the basics – bodyweight exercises that stressed movement. Sure I did my share of pumping iron but nothing to the extreme. I am currently in my early 50's and to this day I've never had to lift hundreds of pounds over my head. On the other hand, I routinely need to bend down, pick things up, twist my body and move about in all different directions. I train for the activities I enjoy, which basically means I train movement. Our bodies were designed to move so training in this way requires very little heavy equipment.

We move in three dimensions yet most gym equipment – certainly the bulk of what you would find at one – moves in only two. This is beginning to change. It's almost a challenge now to find a city park without a boot camp style workout going on. Obstacle Course and Mud Runs are now almost a weekly event. Even the oldest of old-school globe-gyms are beginning to carve out small "functional areas", yet I feel much of the fitness industry does far less than it should in supporting or encouraging this type of training.

Functional exercises incorporate multiple joints and muscles. Instead of only moving the elbows, for example, a functional exercise might involve the elbows, shoulders, spine, hips, knees and ankles. Introducing this type of training and applying it properly into a training regimen can make everyday activities easier and improve quality of life while reducing risk of injury.

As we age the combined effects of increasingly sedentary lifestyles and lifestyle choices tend to add up. Balance, muscle strength, agility and overall functionality lead to increased chance of falling and injury. Proper functional training goes a long way toward reducing risks and maintaining optimal performance for as long as possible.

I feel that I am in my best shape yet – certainly better than I was at 40 or even 30 years old. While I cannot (more accurately I choose not to) lift quite as much dead weight as the 25 year old personal trainers and assorted muscle-heads at the gym I can most certainly keep up with or even exceed many of them when it comes to stamina and the more intense interval-type training sessions. I attribute this primarily to bodyweight exercises that have turned the body into a machine. I train as I live - in all three dimensions - and therefore I utilize muscles all along the kinetic chain. Best of all, I very seldom get hurt training this way, and I tend to bounce back very quickly on the rare occasion when pain or an injury does flair up.

While there are many benefits to training functionally the only downside I can really put a finger on – and to be honest I don't consider it a downside at all - is that it's not designed to bulk up the musculature. Now I've never really had a desire to look quite so freakishly huge as some of the people I see at the gym. You know what I'm talking about, right? The ones who repeatedly lift the entire stack of weights with less than optimal form and then slam them down so everyone else can be impressed.

Functional workouts serve a dual purpose. It is very simple to combine resistance training and cardiovascular exercises along all three planes of movement. They are also very time-efficient. There is really very little need for bulky or expensive equipment. Going to the gym becomes optional as they can be done at home or anywhere. Functional training is simple to do and great for just about anyone at any age.

Functional training is, in my opinion, one of the most efficient ways to train, and the results come quickly. These workouts are designed to increase your metabolic rate. In so doing your body burns more calories throughout the entire day. In short you can burn fat very quickly.

As these workouts focus on movement across all three planes of motion it is amazing just how quickly core strength improves. The core is actually made up of roughly 30 muscles. Body weight exercises are capable of improving all of them while also improving balance, flexibility and range of motion.

One of the main reasons people don't stick with a fitness regimen is boredom. They know a few basic exercises that appear to hit the main muscle groups and that's all they ever do. In short order they dread having to go to the same place at the same time to do the same thing over and over again. Functional training, as I said, is training for the way you move. Just about anything that incorporates normal healthy movement patters will do the trick. There are hundreds of ways to mix things up to ensure that boredom is never an issue. They can be done alone or as part of a group, together or as a competition.

With an aging population and increasing demands on our time exercising in this way is the safest, most efficient and effective way I know to get fit, stay fit and perform at optimal levels.

Pillar #3
Activate Cellular Pathways

"It's what we think we know that keeps us from learning."

~ Claude Bernard

There is nothing more frustrating than a closed mind. It keeps us stuck in the past, and from a healthcare perspective the past is where we don't want to be. For that matter the present is not much better. In terms of healthcare I believe we must set our sights on the future, for that is where healthcare becomes WellCare. WellCare, as I define it, is wellness from the inside out. It is activating our bodies so that they heal themselves naturally. The future, as I see it, is here now. Open your minds and you will see it right before your eyes.

ANTIOXIDANTS WE TAKE VS. ANTIOXIDANTS WE MAKE

At the center of Cellular Health, as I see it, are the very capabilities of the cells in our bodies. Ever since I can remember the mantra of healthcare has been Antioxidants and vitamins. Multivitamins and vitamin supplements have been the solution. As a child I remember my mother pumping me full of orange juice and vitamin C tablets whenever I got sick. When I got out on my own my get-well regimen included as much vitamin C as I could stomach for a couple days. By then I would feel better – or the cold would have run its course.

Science is evolving and we now know much more about how our bodies work naturally as well as how they react to medications and supplements. For example, I'll bet no more than one or two people out of every 100 currently know that our bodies are capable of manufacturing our own antioxidants, and that the antioxidants our bodies make are significantly more powerful and effective at neutralizing free radical damage than are the direct antioxidants we invest through diet and vitamin supplements. Scientists have been studying this for years now. We know it to be true, and yet we remain stuck in this "old school" mindset that we must take antioxidant supplements in order to get and remain healthy.

Personally I enjoy foods that are known to be rich in antioxidants and I eat them nearly every day. As delicious as these foods are – and I believe we should be including them in our daily meals – they are all considered to be "direct antioxidants" which means they offset the free radicals in our cells at a 1 to 1 rate. In reality, activating this Nrf2 pathway in our bodies has been clinically proven to be much more effective. This creates "indirect antioxidants" in the body that can offset free radicals at a rate of approximately 1 million to one. There is a book, *Deadly Antioxidants* that addresses this matter in detail. I've included a brief excerpt below.

"Scientists have known for many years that high doses of isolated nutrients can actually cause more problems than they prevent. Recent examples are beta- carotene in smokers (leading to more lung cancer) and vitamin C in cancer patients (which protects cancer cells more effectively than it does

healthy cells). The "take-away" message from such studies is not that antioxidant vitamins are always "bad" – but rather that synthetic, isolated, high-dose antioxidant supplements are bad."

"The idea of 'making antioxidants' (naturally within our cells) compared to the standard approach of 'taking antioxidants' (in the form of high-dose vitamin supplements) is a fundamentally-different approach to protecting the body from oxidative stress."

"At the very center of this cellular protective pathway is a protein called 'Nrf2' that serves as a 'master regulator' of the body's antioxidant response. You might think of Nrf2 as a 'thermostat' within our cells that senses the level of oxidative stress and other stressors and turns on internal protective mechanisms."

We have the ability to access this "Master Regulator" of antioxidants. In doing do we can significantly reduce the level of oxidative stress and cellular damage in our bodies. As I said before, pharmaceutical companies are all over this science and they are actively seeking out synthetic methods of activating this Nrf2 pathway. While I believe this to be a step in a positive direction I also know that many of these synthetic compounds come with side effects and that some of these side effects are frightening at best and potentially deadly at their worst. One of the issues I've been able to identify is that the synthetic compounds out there today activate the Nrf2 Pathway by simply turning it on like a fire hose, and that's not how the body works naturally. In actuality this pathway turns itself on and off as needed, which is why approaching this with natural ingredients and formulations has been proven to be safer and more effective than the synthetic formulations out there.

Also, pharmaceuticals are developed to treat specific diseases - Cancer, MS, Diabetes... Simple logic dictates that if the Nrf2 Pathway is the master regulator of antioxidants in the body then activating it would benefit all people in every area of the body. Fortunately there ARE natural ways to activate this pathway and significantly reduce the damage caused by the never-ending assault of free radicals.

One of these more natural ways to activate Nrf2 is through diet. Remember from earlier that these are the direct antioxidants that offset free radicals on a 1:1 basis and are other more effective ways to activate Nrf2 in the body. That said this is still sound advice and clean, healthy foods to be eating on a regular basis.

Here is a partial list of commonly found food sources that contain nutrients known to help activate the Nrf2 pathway:

Fruits: Red and purple grapes, apples, red, blue and purple berries, citrus fruits and juices - especially oranges, grapefruits and lemons.

Red wine

Teas: green, white, black and oolong

Dark chocolate

Vegetables: yellow onions, scallions, kale, Brussels sprouts, cauliflower and broccoli are especially good for this, as are celery, hot peppers and green beans

Herbs: Parsley and thyme

Legumes: soy beans and other soy products, green beans, chick peas and mung beans

There are dozens of delicious ways to incorporate these ingredients into your meal plans. You might enjoy them so much that you'll forget they are good for you.

Pillar #4
Heal from Within

"Natural forces within us are the true healers of disease."

~ Hippocrates

DONNA'S STORY: "I WAS SKEPTICAL..."

"When I had some pain near the ball of my foot, I tried all the normal things you are supposed to do -- icing, ibuprofen, rest. Days later and it was still bothering me. Rick said 'Let me do a treatment on it.' I was skeptical. After all, how could a little wand rubbed up and down my foot for 15 minutes really help? Well, was I wrong! After just one treatment the pain was nearly gone--like it never existed! I don't know how it works, I just know it does. (Actually, Rick gave me more description of what's going on at the cellular level and healing, so he's better at explaining the details of how it works than I am.) What I was most happy about, though, was the speed with which this painless treatment worked. I highly recommend Rick to treat the aches and pains you may have."

~ Donna Kozik
Accomplished Author, Coach and
"40-something beginning boxer"

BEV - "THIS RATES AS SOME OF THE BEST..."

"Recently I took tumble down a stair case and, while no serious injuries, I was extremely sore the next day. After this happened and I got home I immediately began icing my right knee and left ankle. It seemed that there was going to be a very large bruise on the top of my foot. The next day I saw Rick at our Rotary meeting limping and grousing in pain. That afternoon he came to my home for the first of two treatments on my ankle and knee. The next morning I was at about 85 percent recovery and the

bruising was almost non-existent. That day we did another treatment and I was at 95 percent pain free the next morning. I have had lots of experience over the years with physical therapy— this rates as some of the best I have had. I strongly recommend this process for soft tissue injuries."

~ Beverly F, San Diego, CA

ACCIDENTS HAPPEN

We can't just live in a bubble. Accidents DO happen and people get injured. Sometimes we need traditional Western medicine to repair the damage. There are other times, however, when there might be a more holistic, safer and less invasive or restricted way to address the issue.

Making smart and educated decisions on which direction to go is to a large degree only possible with an open mind. Health insurers and healthcare systems have their take on how you should be receiving care and sometimes they are absolutely correct. Sometimes, however, there may be options requiring less pain, less downtime, fewer risks and lower costs yet are equally if not more effective than the traditional Western Medicine route. Unless we are willing to open our minds and explore options – some of which aren't covered by insurance because our insurance carriers haven't yet recognized these modalities – we will elongate the pain and the healing process.

To illustrate, dial-up internet is now pretty much a thing of the past. The rotary dial telephone is a relic as well. Ask a Millennial to describe a Rolodex and I'll bet they would look at you clueless. My point is that technology has evolved. Medicine has evolved. Just about everything has evolved, yet minds remain closed.

I have a business partner who is a very prominent physician in a very prestigious hospital. He explained to me once the thought process of doctors and medical professionals like himself. When he was first exposed to the idea that by activating pathways in our bodies we can effectively reduce the root cause of several diseases prevalent today he quickly dismissed it. He was, after all, a doctor. He studied. He went to medical school. He was at the top of his game. If he didn't know about it then it simply wasn't true.

It reminded me of a joke I heard a long time ago. There's a long, long line of people waiting to get into Heaven. Way back at the very end of the line a little old man with a big grey beard starts pushing his way to the front. He's pushing and mumbling and cutting in front of everyone while shouting "Out of the way. I'm a doctor!" Well, the little old man finally gets to the front of the line and shouts "Open the gate. I'm a doctor!" The sentry at the gate opens the gate and the little old man marches through and out of sight. The people in line were all confused at this and began to complain to the sentry. "Why does he get to cut in line? Who does he think he is?" To which the sentry explained "Oh, that's God. He just THINKS he's a doctor."

Anyway, back to my colleague, the doctor. After

repeated attempts by his wife and others to research this area he finally began to look into it. Once he did he began to realize there was real actual science behind it. Doctors revere independent peer-reviewed research studies. That was what opened the door to his eventual endorsement and involvement. Essentially by that point it was his idea all along.

My point is that it IS possible to open a mind – even one as tightly closed as a doctor's. It takes time though, and if by sharing my experience I can help others cut to the chase and just be more open and receptive from the start then I can help to improve the lives and the healing process for many, many people.

Non-Surgical, Drug-Free Pain Treatment Options

The following are examples of non-surgical, drug free pain treatment options available today.

CORRECTIVE EXERCISE

A systematic process of identifying a neuromusculoskeletal dysfunction, developing a plan of action, and implementing an integrated corrective strategy. This modality can help to minimize pain and restore range of motion. This involves an assessment to identify muscular imbalances followed by a four-part process to relax and stretch overactive muscles, strengthen and activate under active muscles and re-integrate normal movement patterns.

MUSCLE MANIPULATION

Manual manipulation of the affected area by applying force to the joints, muscles, and ligaments.

BEHAVIOR MODIFICATION

I see this method as pain management more so than pain treatment. There is no question that relaxation, meditation and the power of the mind to control muscle tension, blood pressure, heart rate and the body's response to pain has been proven to be effective. There are many benefits to these types of behavior modification and cognitive therapies, but mainly they address the symptoms as opposed to the root cause of many types of pain and functionality.

HEAT AND ICE THERAPY

The age-old thinking of hot and cold packs to superficially heat or cool the skin still exists. In many of these cases quicker and more effective results can be achieved by, as I continue to preach, activating the body at the cellular level to simply "re-connect" neural pathways to the brain in order to stimulate the body to repair itself. If this can be done immediately upon these injuries - before cell function begins to shut down - pain can be significantly reduced or even eliminated altogether, and healing can be close to immediate.

ELECTROTHERAPY

The most commonly known type of electrotherapy is transcutaneous electrical nerve stimulation (TENS) that seeks to minimize pain by means of a low-voltage electrical stimulation that interacts with the sensory nervous system. The issue with TENS therapy is the steady signal that hits the skin. This regularity of this signal is often recognized by the body as a potential threat. This causes the cells to protect themselves, which means the signal is not reaching its intended destination. While it feels good while undergoing treatment, it is nowhere near as effective as it should be given its popularity.

SCENAR

Earlier we introduced the term "Homeostasis". Once again, homeostasis is defined as the tendency of the body to seek and maintain a condition of balance or equilibrium within its internal environment, even when faced with external changes. Every function of our bodies communicates harmoniously in order to maintain a homeostatic state.

Normal healthy tissue has a low-level electrical field associated with it. When there is a trauma or an injury this field becomes disrupted and some of the cell functions shut down. This is where the pain and inflammation associated with such injuries stem. Simply put, SCENAR treatments help to restore this electrical field to normal. The aim of a SCENAR treatment is to stimulate the body's own healing powers by emitting an electromagnetic signal that is almost identical to the human nerve signal. Because it mirrors what happens naturally in the body the cells don't shift into self-protection mode like they do with other modalities. This signal travels along special types of nerve fibers to the brain, which activates the cells at the mitochondrial level resulting in the production of neuropeptides to rapidly advance healing. When applied to the point of pain, the brain also releases endorphins, which are the body's own powerful pain relieving substances.

SCENAR treatment is an entirely non-invasive biofeedback modality. There are no drugs or surgery involved. The SCENAR device is placed directly on the skin, where it collects electromagnetic signals that are modified and sent back to the body. This biofeedback is what distinguishes it from TENS machines and other electrical therapies. It is particularly beneficial in reducing pain and inflammation and in the acceleration of healing soft tissue injuries. Many people feel an improved sense of well-being and better sleeping patterns following their treatments. While not currently well known in the USA, it is widely used by many world class athletes and sports teams in the treatment of a variety of injuries and ailments.

REACH BEYOND YOURSELF

One extra piece of the puzzle, and one I will include here in the fourth pillar, is to think and act beyond oneself. By this I mean having - as Rotary International puts it - a "Service Above Self" mindset. Take a few minutes each day to positively and unselfishly impact someone else's life. This can be as simple as holding open a door, giving someone a compliment or a simple "hello" to a perfect stranger. Do it because it's a nice thing to do and not because you want something from them in return. Something happens when we do something nice for another with no expectations. It spreads a little joy. It makes the world a better place. It may start a chain reaction of positive deeds. There are even tales of kindnesses that came at just the right moment so as to actually prevent a crime or a suicide attempt. Go ahead and give it a try. It may even make you feel better yourself.

Conclusion

"It isn't bragging if you can do it"

~ Dizzy Dean

I've been called a lot of things in my life. One thing I've tried hard never to be is boastful. I have always been a man of my word and I pride myself on my integrity. If I say I will do something I do it. If I say I can do something it means I really can do it. Hence the quote at the beginning of this chapter by former Major League pitcher Dizzy Dean, "It isn't bragging if you can do it." What I do works. Activating the body's Nrf2 Pathway works. Lowering oxidative stress in the body works. Triggering cells at the mitochondrial level to produce the chemicals the body needs to heal itself works. The way I train my clients works. The combination of all that I do REALLY, REALLY works, and it can work for you, too.

WHAT IF...

...Nrf2 ***REALLY IS*** the master regulator of the total antioxidant system?

...the FDA ***REALLY IS*** all about the money?

...healthcare providers and insurance companies ***REALLY DO*** value profits over people?

...as Washington State University states - we ***REALLY ARE*** "... on the verge of a new literature on health effects of Nrf2 which may become the most extraordinary therapeutic and most extraordinary preventative breakthrough in the history of medicine."

...you ignore the rapidly evolving research only to find yourself and your loved ones left behind?

...even half of the recent research findings are true?

WHAT IF?

FINAL THOUGHTS

First of all I'm not here to tell people what to do. I am merely offering up a potential alternative. I believe that by following this protocol myself I am healthier, have more energy, less pain, more functionality, a clearer mind and significantly lower oxidative stress than the majority of the population. I can also state that there have been many, many people who look, feel and perform significantly better for having worked with me. I am convinced this is because of the Four Pillars.

As I am not considered a medical practitioner I need to be very careful how I phrase things. I am in no way making any medical claims here. I am not saying that non-surgical treatments, non-pharmaceutical supplements, rebalancing your metabolism or activating the Nrf2 pathway in your body is going to treat, cure, mitigate or in any way help you. That said, you wouldn't be reading this book unless you were seeking a better, more holistic and possibly more effective way to achieve better health, increased energy, eliminate pain or in some way improve quality of life. And you wouldn't have made it all the way to the end if you weren't at least somewhat convinced what I've said has merit.

Those who follow my "Four Pillars" protocol of eating healthy, training functionally, activating cellular pathways and healing from within are a steadily growing segment of the population. I'd like to say it's beginning to look like a movement, and as movements begin to grow they have a way of influencing change. Any changes we can make to get ourselves back on track, to once again value people over profits and to holistically look, feel and perform at our optimal level are worthwhile changes indeed.

Medical Disclaimer

Always consult your physician before beginning any exercise program. This general information is not intended to diagnose any medical condition or to replace your healthcare professional. Consult with your healthcare professional to design an appropriate exercise prescription. If you experience any pain or difficulty with these exercises, stop and consult your healthcare provider. If you experience any symptoms of weakness, unsteadiness, light-headedness or dizziness, chest pain or pressure, nausea, or shortness of breath. Mild soreness after exercise may be experienced after beginning a new exercise. Contact your physician if the soreness does not improve after 3-4 days

The information contained in this book has not been evaluated by the Food and Drug Administration (FDA). The Information found on this website should not be used to diagnose, cure, prevent or mitigate disease. This website is provided for educational purposes only. Statements contained herein are presented in an effort to share information about free radical biology , medicinal foods and advances in nutrition only. Content may change frequently and may be incomplete; consequently, information presented herein may not be accurate until finalized. Dietary supplement research and information expressed herein should be considered anecdotal in nature or opinions and hypotheses rather than generally accepted science. Unless otherwise noted, the studies presented herein

www.ingramcontent.com/pod-product-compliance
Lightning Source LLC
Chambersburg PA
CBHW072200280526
45788CB00002B/817